MUDRAS & MEDITATION
— for —
CHAKRA HEALING

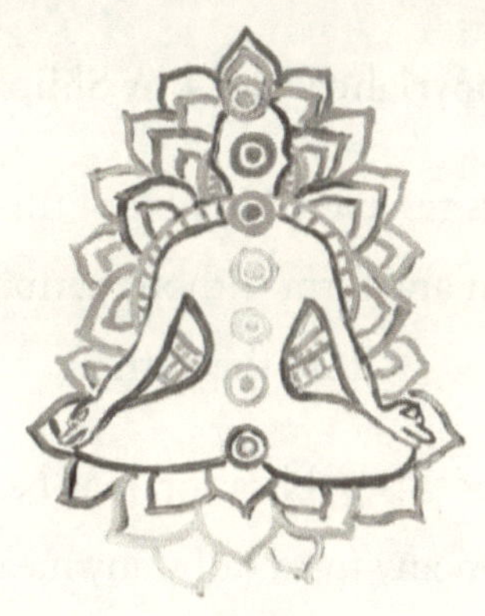

*Boost Your Energy, Reduce Stress, Find Clarity, and
Experience a Lasting Sense of Inner Peace*

By

SHILPA MEHTA

PREFACE

In this book, we embark on a transformative journey through the realms of Mudras, Chakras, and Meditation—a journey that aims to harmonize mind, body, and soul. Whether you are new to these ancient practices or seeking a deeper connection, this guide offers a gentle yet profound exploration of how to activate and balance the energy centers within you.

Mudras, often described as sacred hand gestures, are much more than symbolic postures. They are gateways to unlocking hidden energies and enhancing our overall well-being. In this book, you will discover how these simple yet powerful hand positions can bring about profound changes in your physical, emotional, and mental states.

Chakras, the energy centers that govern different aspects of our being, lie at the core of our vitality. By understanding each chakra, from the Mooladhara, the root of stability, to the Sahasrara, the crown of consciousness, we begin to recognize how these centers influence our daily lives. Visualizing and activating these chakras is a path to realizing the potential that lies within each of us.

Meditation ties together the elements of Mudras and Chakras, guiding our awareness inward and allowing us to cultivate a state of balance and clarity. Each meditation in this book is specifically designed to activate and harmonize the energy of a particular chakra, providing a step-by-step approach to achieving inner equilibrium.

Throughout this book, you will find thoughtfully illustrated drawings of each chakra and the corresponding mudra, making it easy to understand and practice the techniques. As you immerse yourself in these practices, may you experience the unfolding of your inner energy, bringing peace, balance, and a deeper sense of self-awareness.

May this journey uplift you, inspire you, and bring you closer to your true self.

DEDICATION

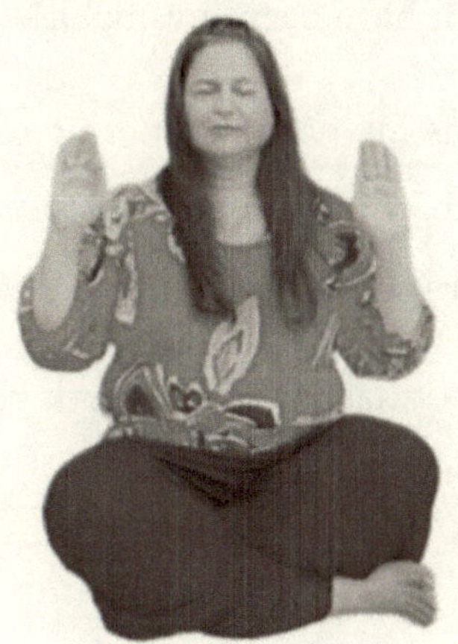

To all educators who ignite minds and nurture hearts—your dedication is the essence of teaching.

To my mentors and colleagues, whose wisdom and support have guided me.

To my students, past and present, whose enthusiasm inspires me daily.

To my daughter Reekta, son-in-law Karan, and grandchildren, whose love and faith in me have been a constant source of strength and joy.

To my sister Trupti, Dr. Rohit Gandhi, and my friend Dr. Sanjivv Gandhi, whose unwavering love and encouragement have been invaluable.

This book is my humble offering to my late mother and Yogi Vinod, whose influence and guidance continue to inspire me.

Your support has made this work possible, and your spirit shines through every page.

Thank you for being a part of this journey and for helping to make this dream a reality.

Special Thanks

*Special thanks to **Ms. Renu Mathur** for her incredible artwork in my books on chakras, meditation, and mudras.*

Her creativity and attention to detail have beautifully brought these concepts to life, enhancing the reading and learning experience for all.

Her artistic vision has added a unique and meaningful touch to these works, and I am deeply grateful for her contribution.

Table Of Contents

★ ★ ★

Introduction To Mudras

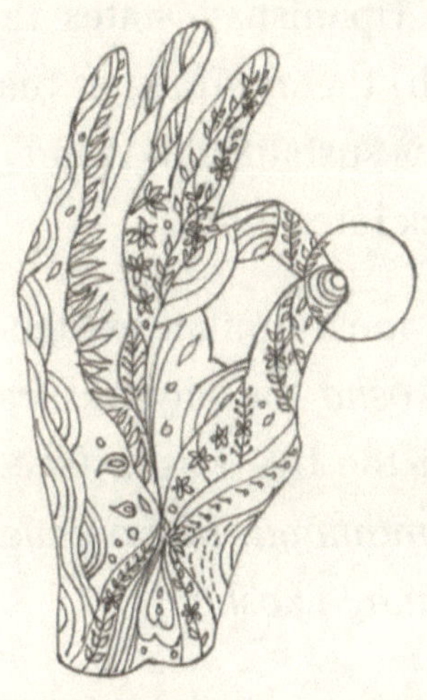

Historically, mudras have been integral to Vedic and Buddhist rituals, with their benefits recognized and utilized for centuries.

Mudras are powerful tools that bridge the connection between the mind and body, helping to

- release energy blockages,

- stimulate the production of endorphins,

- elevate mood,

- and boost overall vitality.

With a profound healing effect on both the physical and mental planes.

Taitteriya Upanishad states the Pancha[five] Kosha[sheath] theory. It states that everything in the universe is sustained by *Anna [food],* and also dissolves back into *Anna.*

The gross most human existence is known as *Annamaya kosha* the physical frame that is the outermost of the five *Koshas[sheaths] the other four are Pranamaya, Manomaya, Vigyanmaya and Anandamaya kosha.*

On a subtler level, mudras facilitate a connection between the Pancha Koshas— specifically the Annamaya (physical), Manomaya (mental), and Pranamaya (energy) sheaths. Regular practice of mudras manipulates Prana (life force energy) in a way that redirects this energy inward, creating protective barriers within the body.

Annamaya Kosha consists of five elements *(Pancha Bhutas),* namely earth *(Prithvi)* (पृथ्वी), water *(Jala* or *Apa)* (जल), fire *(Agni* or *Tejas)* (तेजस),

wind *(Vayu)* (वायु), and space *(Akash)* (आकाश). It is nourished by the gross food that we consume.

Each of the five fingers corresponds to one of the five basic elements, allowing specific hand mudras to enhance and purify the chakras. Mudras serve as a powerful tool to harmonize these five elements, thereby strengthening the pranic system and fuelling our aspiration for higher levels of consciousness.

Types of Mudras: An Overview

Mudras are powerful gestures designed to serve various purposes, from promoting healing to enhancing meditation and spiritual growth. Here's a brief overview of the main categories:

1. **Healing Mudras:** The body's five elements—earth, water, fire, air, and ether can be restored by practising the Healing mudras. It focuses on restoring physical, emotional, and mental well-being by balancing the five elements. The body's natural healing processes can be enhanced by these mudras alleviating ailments and boosting immunity. Prana Mudra helps

revitalize the body and strengthen life force, while Apan Mudra is known for its purifying effects on toxins.

2. **Chakra Mudras:** The energy centers, or chakras can get activated, balanced, and aligned by practising these Mudras. Each chakra governs specific aspects of the body and consciousness, and these mudras help clear blockages, enhancing the flow of energy. Like, Prithvi Mudra associated with the root chakra (Muladhara), helps promote grounding and stability, like Anahata Mudra connects with the heart chakra (Anahata), fostering love, empathy, and emotional balance.

3. **Meditation Mudras:** Focusing the mind, channeling energy, and enhancing inner awareness, the integral meditative experiences are deepened by practising the Meditation mudras. States of calm, concentration, and spiritual connection are also strengthened *Dhyana Mudra*, is a great example of meditation mudras, and it is often depicted in statues of Buddha,

symbolizing serenity and inner peace. while Chin Mudra aids in mental clarity and spiritual awakening.

Each category of mudras offers distinct benefits, allowing practitioners to choose those that align with their specific needs and goals, supporting holistic health, spiritual development, and personal growth.

The right way to practice Mudras

Mudras involve gently touching the thumb to different fingers in specific positions, with light pressure and relaxed hands. Initially, it may be challenging to maintain the mudra as fingers and hands can tire or slip out of position, especially if there are pranic imbalances in the body. These imbalances often manifest in the hands, making it difficult to hold the mudra. However, with regular practice the prana begins to flow more smoothly, increasing flexibility in the hands and fingers, making it easier. With consistent practice and determination, any physical or mental resistance can be overcome, and the corresponding regions of the body and mind can be healed through mudra practice. Mudras are most effective when practiced during meditation or in a mindful, calm state.

Each mudra has a unique impact, targeting specific connections and influencing unconscious reflexes and ingrained habits. To experience the full benefits, mudras should be held for 10-15 minutes and practiced regularly, making them particularly effective during a 20-minute meditation session.

The right posture to practice Mudras

Mudras can be practiced in any position, whether seated on a chair, lying down, standing, or even walking. Regardless of the posture, it's important to practice them symmetrically and in a centered position to ensure the body remains stable and relaxed. While mudras are effective in any body posture, the ideal position is seated with the spine and head aligned in a straight line. Muscle tension should be minimal, just enough to maintain the posture. The mind should be calm and focused, with attention to deep, smooth, and serene breathing to achieve the best results from the mudras.

Generally, mudras can be practiced by anyone and have few contraindications. However, because they are advanced practices that can stimulate and awaken Prana, Chakras, and Kundalini energy, it's recommended to learn them under the guidance of an experienced teacher, especially when starting.

The meditations in this book are designed with this in mind, making them simple and suitable for beginners.

Introduction to Chakras

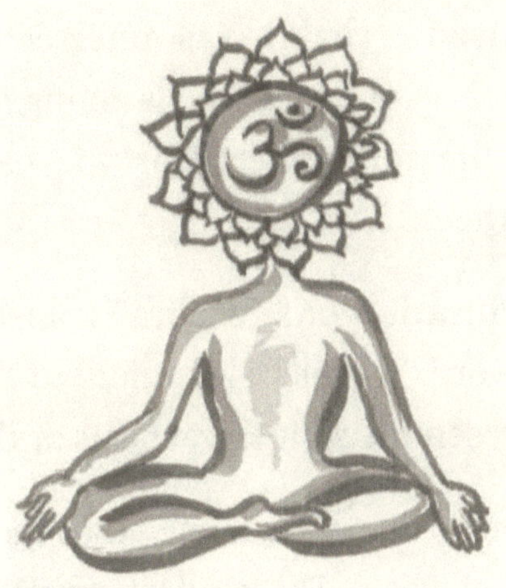

According to yoga, you are so much more than just your physical body (*sthula sarira*). You also have a subtle, energy body (*sukshma sarira*). This energy body is made up of subtle energy pathways through which the life force flows. There are certain points in the body where these energy pathways converge, and you guessed it, these energy centers are called chakras. Chakras correspond to nerve plexuses in the physical body.

While it is believed that the human body contains 109 chakras, seven are considered the most significant. These seven main chakras are interconnected by subtle energy pathways, allowing life force energy to flow throughout the body. Imagine chakras as intersections where roads meet, with the channels acting as the roads and the life force energy as the cars moving, through them.

The Sanskrit word "chakra" translates to the English word "wheel." This refers to the way that chakras resemble spinning wheels or discs.

The chakras are among the most famous concepts of yoga. The earliest written record of chakras comes from the Vedas, which are ancient Indian texts that describe the philosophy of yoga. The precise age of the Vedas is unknown, but they are thousands of years old. Evidence of chakras, spelled cakra, is also found in the Shri Jabala Darshana Upanishad, the Cudamini Upanishad, the Yoga-Shikka Upanishad and the Shandilya Upanishad. It was an integral part of Tantric yoga traditions later adopted by one sect of Buddhism called Vajrayana. Vajrayana, often referred to as Tantric Buddhism, is a form of Buddhism that evolved in India and spread to regions like Tibet.

It incorporates secret practices similar to those in Tantra Yoga, including asceticism, specific body postures, and mystical rituals.

Beliefs differ between the Indian religions, with many Buddhist texts consistently mentioning four or five chakras, while Hindu sources reference six or seven. Other traditions hold that there are thousands of energy centers but a few are the most important. The lack of a universally accepted standard has led to variation and diversity in the interpretation and understanding of chakras. Several sects within Hinduism have their unique interpretations and understandings of the concept of chakras. Here are some of the major sects that have different perspectives on chakras:

- Bhakti Yoga: In Bhakti Yoga, the number of chakras varies, but the focus is often on the heart chakra as the center of spiritual devotion.

- Ayurveda (3): In Ayurveda, there are three main chakras, known as the "Marmas," which are considered to be the focal points of the physical, mental, and spiritual energies in the body.

- Shaivism (5): In Shaivism, there are five chakras, with the focus being on the heart and crown chakras.

- Tantra (6): In Tantra, there are traditionally said to be four to six chakras, with the crown chakra being considered the highest.

- Kashmir Shaivism (6-7): In Kashmir Shaivism, there are six or seven chakras, with the focus being on the awakening of the divine energy within.

- Hatha Yoga (7): In Hatha Yoga, there are seven main chakras, but some Hatha Yoga traditions also recognize additional chakras.

- Kundalini Yoga (7): In Kundalini Yoga, there are seven main chakras, but additional minor chakras are also recognized.

- Nath Tradition (8): In the Nath tradition, there are eight main chakras, with the emphasis being on the awakening of the divine energy through these centers.

- Vaishnavism (12): In Vaishnavism, there are twelve chakras, with the emphasis being on the spiritual ascent through these centers.

Early Sanskrit texts describe chakras both as meditative visualizations, often depicted as flowers and combined with mantras, and as subtle energy points within the body. Each of the seven main chakras is symbolized by a lotus or different types of flowers. This floral imagery represents the delicate, refined state of consciousness experienced during deep meditation, where the mind becomes vibrant, alive, and fresh, akin to a blossoming flower. In this heightened state of awareness, one can sense the awakening and movement of energy within the system.

- Chakras serve as focal points in various ancient meditation practices, particularly those rooted in Tantra. In Kundalini Yoga, specific techniques—such as pranayama (breathing exercises), visualizations, mudras (hand gestures), bandhas (body locks), kriyas (purification practices), and mantras (sacred sounds)—are employed to influence and direct the flow of subtle energy through the chakras.

- Positioned along the spinal column, from the base of the spine to the crown of the head, chakras are conceptualized as centers of energy rather than as physical entities with definite nervous nodes or precise physical locations. In tantric systems, chakras are envisioned as ever-present and significant, serving as channels for psychic and emotional energy within the body.

- To better understand this, imagine your body as having a complex network of circuits. In the physical body, this network is made up of arteries, veins, nerves, and the organs they connect to. In addition to this physical circuitry, yogis of ancient times described a subtle or energy body that cannot be seen or touched. This subtle body is where all life-force energy flows, and it comprises chakras (energy centers) and nadis (energy channels). Unlike the physical body, which consists of visible, tangible mass, the subtle body is made up of invisible energy, encompassing both the mind and emotions. The energy or spiritual state of the subtle body directly influences the physical body, and vice versa. This interplay means that the condition of a person's chakras can significantly impact their overall health and well-being.

The Evolution of the Western Chakra System

The modern "Western chakra system" began to take shape in the late 19th century, heavily influenced by various esoteric traditions. It started with H. P. Blavatsky and other Theosophists in the 1880s and was further developed through Sir John Woodroffe's 1919 book, *The Serpent Power*, and Charles W. Leadbeater's 1927 book, *The Chakras*. As time went on, the system expanded to include psychological attributes, rainbow colors, and a myriad of correspondences with other esoteric frameworks, such as alchemy, astrology, gemstones, homeopathy, Kabbalah, and Tarot.

While these adaptations made the ancient wisdom of chakras more accessible to a broader audience, they also introduced numerous misconceptions. Originally, knowledge about chakras was a closely guarded science, reserved for sincere practitioners deeply committed to their spiritual journey. As this knowledge became more widely disseminated, it sparked greater public interest and exploration in spiritual practices, but it also led to the spread of dubious theories—such as the notion that eating foods of certain colors can activate corresponding chakras.

This evolution reflects how the Western understanding of chakras has diverged from its original roots. The contemporary view of the human energy field often draws from fragmented interpretations that emerged during the New Age movement, selectively borrowing from various spiritual traditions. The popular seven-chakra system has become so ubiquitous that even those with little spiritual inclination recognize it. Over time, this system has been associated with specific colors, crystals, attributes, and scents—many of which differ significantly from the traditional Vedic and Yogic understandings.

However, despite these distortions, there is a positive aspect to this evolution. Even through fragmented interpretations, these adaptations have sparked curiosity and interest in spiritual concepts that might otherwise have remained obscure. Consider this analogy: Just as light passing through a prism reveals a spectrum of seven colours, our understanding of the chakras, including their shapes, forms, and colours, helps us navigate the material world. To transcend from the material to the spiritual, a process similar to sunlight refracting through raindrops to create a rainbow is needed—this rainbow reveals the true nature of light.

In this analogy, materialism is like cloudy days that obscure the sunlight, requiring us to seek illumination to grasp the essence of light. Yogic sadhana (spiritual practice) enables us to move beyond these limitations, leading to an understanding of light in its purest form. As we progress through the chapters dedicated to each of the seven chakras, the aim is to guide you toward a state beyond colours and attributes—where you can adapt seamlessly to any situation, becoming like clear light.

Just as gemstones such as emeralds, rubies, and sapphires, known for their vibrant colors of green, red, and blue, are not inherently coloured but appear so due to the interaction of light with their structure, you too can learn to blend effortlessly with your surroundings. When placed against a blue background, you reflect blue; against a red background, you reflect red. By transcending the refracted light and embracing a reflective state, you attain a clearer and more profound vision.

Introduction To Meditation

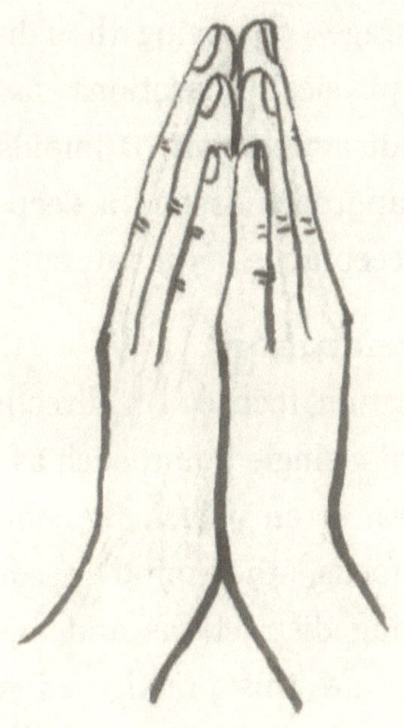

Principles of Meditation

Meditation is a profound practice designed to cultivate mental clarity, emotional balance, and spiritual awareness. At its core, meditation involves training the mind to focus, be present, and observe thoughts and emotions without judgment. While there are various forms and techniques, several foundational principles guide all meditation practices:

- **Mindfulness:** This principle emphasizes bringing complete attention to the present moment. Mindfulness meditation encourages observing thoughts, emotions, and physical sensations as they arise, without attachment or impulsive reaction. This approach fosters a deeper awareness and acceptance of the present.

- **Concentration:** Concentration meditation focuses on directing the mind toward a single point, such as the breath, a mantra, or an object. By concentrating on this focus, the mind becomes calmer, reducing distractions and mental chatter. Over time, this practice enhances mental discipline and clarity.

- **Breath Awareness:** The breath is a natural anchor in meditation, linking the mind and body. By focusing on the rhythm of breathing, practitioners can calm the nervous system, relax the body, and reach a deeper meditative state. Breath awareness also supports mindfulness and concentration.

- **Non-Attachment:** This principle teaches practitioners to observe thoughts and experiences without becoming emotionally entangled. Non-attachment does not mean indifference but rather cultivating the ability to experience life with equanimity and inner peace, free from the chaos of attachment.

- **Inner Stillness:** Many meditation practices aim to achieve a state of inner stillness or silence. This state is marked by a profound sense of peace and presence that goes beyond the mind's typical fluctuations. In this stillness, practitioners experience a deeper connection with their true self and the world around them.

Techniques/Types of Meditation

Meditation is a versatile practice with many techniques, each offering unique benefits and catering to different needs. Here are some of the most popular meditation techniques:

- **Mindfulness Meditation:** This practice involves paying attention to the present moment, observing thoughts, sensations, and emotions without judgment. Practitioners focus on their breath or another anchor, gently redirecting their attention whenever the mind wanders. Mindfulness meditation is widely practiced for stress reduction, emotional regulation, and enhanced self-awareness.

- **Concentration Meditation:** Concentration meditation focuses the mind on a single object, sound, or thought. Common examples include focusing on a candle flame, repeating a mantra (like "Om"), or visualizing a specific image. This technique strengthens mental focus, improves attention span, and helps quiet the mind.

- **Guided Visualization:** Visualization meditation involves creating mental images to evoke a sense of peace, healing, or inspiration. Practitioners may visualize serene landscapes, healing light, or achieving personal goals. This technique can enhance relaxation, boost creativity, and support personal growth by engaging the power of imagination.

- **Loving-Kindness Meditation (Metta):** This technique involves cultivating compassion and love by silently repeating phrases such as "May I be happy, may I be healthy, may I be safe." Practitioners extend these wishes to others, including loved ones, acquaintances, and even those with whom they have conflicts. Loving-kindness meditation fosters empathy, reduces negative emotions, and enhances emotional well-being.

- **Body Scan Meditation:** In body scan meditation, practitioners systematically focus on different parts of the body, from the toes to the head, noticing sensations, tension, or discomfort. This practice promotes relaxation, increases body awareness, and helps release physical and emotional tension.

- **Chakra Meditation:** This technique focuses on the body's energy centers, or chakras. Practitioners visualize the chakras as spinning wheels of light, each with its own color and frequency, working on balancing and energizing them. Chakra meditation enhances emotional balance, spiritual growth, and overall vitality by harmonizing the body's energy system.

- **Transcendental Meditation (TM):** Transcendental Meditation involves silently repeating a mantra provided by a trained instructor to transcend ordinary thought processes and reach a state of deep inner peace and relaxation. TM is known for reducing stress, enhancing creativity, and improving overall well-being.

- **Zen Meditation (Zazen):** Rooted in Zen Buddhism, Zazen involves seated meditation with a focus on the breath and maintaining an upright posture. Practitioners observe thoughts and sensations without attachment, cultivating a sense of awareness and insight. Zen meditation emphasizes discipline, simplicity, and spiritual awakening.

- **Vipassana Meditation:** Vipassana, meaning "insight" or "clear seeing," is one of the oldest meditation techniques from

India. It involves observing thoughts and bodily sensations systematically to gain insight into the nature of reality and the impermanence of all things. This deeply transformative practice fosters self-awareness and liberation from suffering.

Benefits of Meditation

Meditation offers a wide range of benefits that enhance physical, mental, emotional, and spiritual well-being:

- **Stress Reduction**: Meditation effectively reduces stress by calming the mind and body, lowering cortisol levels, and promoting relaxation. Regular practice helps individuals manage stress more effectively, contributing to a balanced and peaceful life.

- **Improved Mental Clarity and Focus**: Meditation enhances cognitive functions like concentration, memory, and mental clarity. It trains the brain to focus on one task at a time, minimizing distractions and increasing productivity.

- **Emotional Balance**: Meditation fosters emotional resilience, allowing practitioners to approach situations with calmness and equanimity. This leads to healthier relationships, a positive outlook, and greater emotional stability.

- **Enhanced Physical Health**: Meditation offers numerous physical health benefits, including lowering blood pressure, boosting immune function, reducing inflammation, and alleviating chronic pain. It also promotes better sleep, enhancing overall health and vitality.

- **Spiritual Growth**: Meditation serves as a profound tool for spiritual development, helping individuals connect with a higher consciousness and a sense of purpose. It facilitates self-discovery, enlightenment, and a deeper understanding of existence.

- **Increased Self-Awareness**: Meditation promotes introspection and self-reflection, enabling individuals to gain deeper insights into their thoughts, behaviours, and motivations. This heightened self-awareness fosters personal growth and a more authentic life.

- **Greater Compassion and Empathy**: Practices like loving-kindness meditation cultivate compassion and empathy, enhancing feelings of interconnectedness and understanding. This promotes kindness, forgiveness, and altruism, fostering more harmonious relationships and communities.

In summary, meditation is a versatile practice that nurtures the mind, body, and spirit.

By exploring its diverse techniques and embracing its wide-ranging benefits, individuals can transform their lives, achieving greater peace, clarity, and fulfilment.

The following chapters will explain how to combine mudras with meditation to amplify their effects.

Each chapter will focus on a specific chakra, detailing the corresponding mudra and meditation technique for that energy center.

Integration Of Mudras With Related Chakra And Meditation

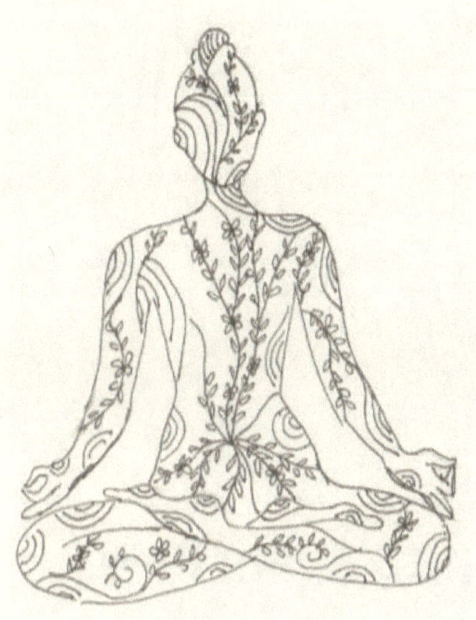

How to Combine Mudras with Meditation for Enhanced Effects

The practice of integrating mudras with meditation combines the subtle energy of hand gestures with the profound focus of meditation. This synergy deepens the meditative experience, balances the body's energy, and enhances overall well-being. Here's a guide to effectively incorporating mudras into your meditation practice:

1. **Choosing the Right Mudra for Your Meditation**

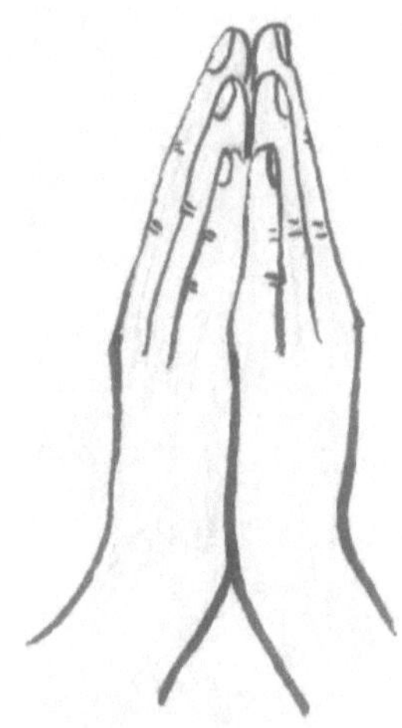

Anjali Mudra

Select a mudra that aligns with your meditation's intention or goal. Different mudras influence the mind and body in unique ways, so choose one that resonates with your needs. For example:

- **Gyan Mudra (Mudra of Knowledge):** Touch the tip of the index finger to the tip of the thumb, with the other fingers extended. This mudra enhances mental clarity and spiritual insight, making it ideal for wisdom-focused meditations.

- **Dhyana Mudra (Meditation Mudra):** Place the right hand on top of the left hand, palms facing up, with the thumbs lightly touching. This mudra symbolizes deep concentration and inner peace, suitable for profound meditative practices.

2. Establishing Your Meditation Posture

Once you've selected the appropriate mudra, establish a comfortable and stable meditation posture:

- **Seated Posture (Sukhasana):** Sit cross-legged with your hands resting on your knees or thighs, holding the chosen mudra. If sitting on a chair, keep your feet flat on the ground and your hands on your lap. Maintain a straight spine and relaxed body.

- **Lying Down (Savasana):** For lying-down meditation, place your hands by your sides with the mudra, palms facing up. This position is ideal for deep relaxation and healing.

3. Focusing Your Attention

With the mudra in place and your posture established, gently close your eyes and bring your attention to your meditation focus, such as your breath, a mantra, or visualization. Allow the mudra to enhance this focus:

- **Breath Awareness:** Notice how the mudra supports the flow of energy with each breath. For example, in Prana Mudra, feel the breath energizing your body and mind.

- **Mantra Meditation:** Repeat your mantra in rhythm with your breath, allowing the mudra to amplify the mantra's effects.

- **Visualization:** Anchor your visualization with the mudra, such as imagining light radiating from your heart center, filling you with compassion and peace.

4. Enhancing Energy Flow and Balance

Mudras influence the body's energy pathways and chakras. Pay attention to the subtle sensations in your hands and fingers and observe how the mudra affects your overall energy.

5. Deepening the Meditative Experience

Allow the mudra to deepen your meditation by reinforcing your intention and focus. The physical touch points of the mudra act as reminders to stay present and influence your mental and emotional state:

- **Cultivating Stillness:** In Dhyana Mudra, focus on the gentle connection of your hands. This symbolizes unity and helps you transcend distractions, entering deep meditation.

- **Opening the Heart:** In Anjali Mudra, bring awareness to the space between your palms at the heart center, expanding your capacity for love and compassion.

- **Awakening Inner Wisdom:** In Gyan Mudra, concentrate on the touch of your index finger and thumb, representing the union of knowledge and wisdom. Allow insights to arise naturally.

6. Concluding the Practice

As you end your meditation, gently release the mudra and take a few moments to observe any shifts in your energy or awareness. Reflect on how the mudra influenced your practice:

- **Expressing Gratitude:** You may bring your hands into Anjali Mudra as a gesture of gratitude for the practice and insights gained.

- **Transitioning Back:** Slowly open your eyes, take deep breaths, and gradually return to your surroundings, carrying a sense of calm and balance into your day.

7. Ongoing Practice and Exploration

The integration of mudras with meditation evolves over, time. As you become more attuned to the subtle energies of mudras, you'll find they can profoundly enhance your meditation practice, bringing greater depth and transformation.

Explore chakra and related mudra meditations to deepen your connection to your inner self, balance your energies, and enhance your well-being.

Feel free to adjust any specific details according to your practice and insights.

Mooladhara (Root) Chakra

The Root of Existence and Stability

Introduction to Mooladhara Chakra

The Mooladhara Chakra, or Root Chakra, is the foundation of our subtle energy body, the source of our most primal energy. The word "Mooladhara" is derived from two Sanskrit words: "Moola," meaning root, and "Adhara," meaning support or base. This chakra is located at the base of the spine, near the perineum, and it is associated with the earth element (Prithvi Tattva). The Mooladhara Chakra governs our sense of security, stability, and survival, acting as the anchor that keeps us grounded in the physical world.

The Mooladhara Chakra is associated with our basic needs, such as food, shelter, and safety. When this chakra is balanced, we feel secure, grounded, and confident in our ability to face life's challenges. However, when it is blocked or imbalanced, we may experience feelings of fear, insecurity, and instability.

Symbolism and Attributes

Mooladhara Chakra / Root Chakra

- **Location:** Base of the spine, near the perineum (between the anus and genitals)

- **Element:** Earth (Prithvi Tattva)

- **Colour:** Deep Red (representing the energy of life and vitality)

- **Shape:** Square (symbolizing stability and groundedness)

- **Petals:** Four (representing the four directions and the foundation of existence)

- **Bija Mantra:** "Lam" (लं)

- **Deity:** Shri Ganesh (the remover of obstacles) and Brahmaji (the creator)

- **Animal Symbol:** Elephant (representing strength, stability, and wisdom)

- **Yantra:** A square with a downward-pointing triangle, symbolizing the grounding energy of the earth

- **Sense:** Smell (associated with the earth element and grounding)

- **Associated Planet:** Mangal, Mars (representing energy, action, and desire)

- **Mudra:** Prithvi Mudra (Earth Mudra)

Mooladhara Chakra in Indian Tradition

In Indian tradition, the Mooladhara Chakra is symbolized by a deep red lotus with four petals, representing the four directions and the foundational nature of this energy center.

In the ancient texts of India, the Mooladhara Chakra is considered the root of our physical and spiritual existence. It is the seat of the Kundalini

Shakti, the divine feminine energy that lies dormant within all beings. This energy, when awakened, rises through the Sushumna Nadi (central energy channel) and activates each chakra, ultimately leading to spiritual enlightenment.

The earth element associated with the Mooladhara Chakra is considered the densest material of all the elements. It represents the physical body, the physical world, and our connection to the natural environment. In Vedic rituals, the earth is honoured as "Bhoomi Devi," the goddess of the earth, and is worshiped for her nurturing and sustaining qualities.

The elephant, the animal symbol of the Mooladhara Chakra, is revered in Indian culture for its strength, patience, and wisdom. Bhagwan Ganesha, who is depicted with the head of an elephant, is the presiding deity of this chakra. He is invoked at the beginning of any new endeavour to remove obstacles and bless the undertaking with success.

Before beginnig the meditation practice, take a moment to learn Prithvi Mudra, a powerful hand gesture associated with the Mooladhara Chakra.

Forming the Mudra

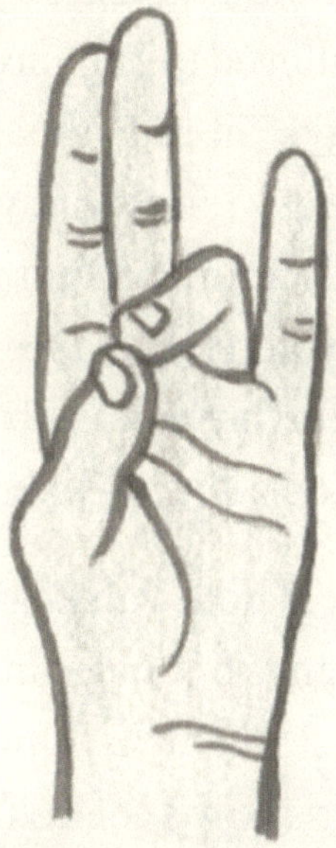

Mooladhara Mudra/Prithvi Mudra (Earth Mudra)

To practice Prithvi Mudra, bring the tip of your ring finger (associated with the earth element) to touch the tip of your thumb. The other three fingers should remain extended and relaxed. This mudra should be practiced with both hands.

Mooladhara Chakra Meditation

Preparation: Begin your practice by choosing a quiet, serene space where you can sit undisturbed. Wear comfortable clothing made from natural fibers like cotton or wool, as these materials are believed to enhance the flow of prana (life force energy). Sit in Padmasana (Lotus Pose) or Sukhasana (Easy Pose) with your back straight. Keep your hands in Anjali Mudra (prayer position) at the centre of your chest. Place a red cloth or mat beneath you to further connect with the grounding energy of the Mooladhara Chakra.

Invocation: Before you begin the meditation, invoke the blessings of Bhagwan Ganesh. You may chant the Ganesh mantra: "Om Gan Ganapataye Namaha" (ॐ गं गणपतये नमः) to seek his guidance and remove any obstacles in your spiritual journey. Visualize his radiant form, with his gentle yet powerful presence, blessing you with stability and protection.

Mudra and Pranayama: Hold Prithvi Mudra with both hands and practice Dirgha Pranayama (Three-Part Breathing) to further enhance your connection to the Mooladhara

Chakra. Inhale deeply, filling your lower abdomen first, then your chest, and finally your upper lungs. With each inhale, visualize yourself drawing in the nurturing energy of the earth. With each exhale, imagine releasing any feelings of insecurity or instability.

Chanting the Bija Mantra: Holding the mudra begin to chant the bija mantra "Lam" (लं) aloud, allowing the sound to resonate in your lower abdomen and pelvis. With each repetition, feel the vibrations awakening and balancing the Mooladhara Chakra.

Visualization of Yantra: Continue chanting, keeping your awareness on the base of your spine. Visualize a deep red lotus with four petals blooming at this point. Imagine it spinning slowly, radiating its grounding energy throughout your body. To further deepen your connection with the Mooladhara Chakra, envision the square yantra of the chakra, stabilizing and balancing your foundation.

Closing the Meditation: As you prepare to conclude, see the Mooladhara Chakra glowing with steady, vibrant energy, spreading warmth and grounding throughout your being. Slowly bring your awareness back to your breath, taking deep, grounding breaths. Gradually open your eyes, taking a moment to feel the effects of the meditation. You may place your palms on the ground and offer a silent prayer of gratitude to Bhoomi Devi for her constant support and sustenance.

Reflecting on the Experience: Consider how you feel in terms of stability, security, and connection to the earth. Take a few moments to reflect on your experience to deepen your understanding of the Mooladhara Chakra and its role in your life.

Benefits of Mooladhara Meditation

- **Physical Well-Being:** Strengthens the lower body, including the legs, feet, and pelvic area. Promotes healthy digestion and elimination.

- **Emotional Stability:** Enhances feelings of security, safety, and confidence. Reduces anxiety, fear, and insecurity.

- **Spiritual Grounding:** Deepens your connection to the earth, grounding your spiritual practices in physical reality. Supports the awakening of Kundalini Shakti.

- **Mental Clarity:** Provides a solid foundation for mental focus and clarity, enabling you to make grounded decisions.

Conclusion

The Mooladhara Chakra is the bedrock of our physical and spiritual existence. By nurturing this chakra through meditation, chanting, mudra practice, and daily grounding activities, we can cultivate a deep sense of security, stability, and connection to the earth. This strong foundation allows us to navigate life's challenges with confidence, knowing that we are supported by the earth's abundant energy. As we balance the Mooladhara Chakra, we lay the groundwork for the awakening of our higher chakras, paving the way for spiritual growth and enlightenment.

Swadhisthana (Sacral) Chakra

The Center of Creativity and Emotional Fluidity

Introduction to Swadhisthana Chakra

The Swadhisthana Chakra, also known as the Sacral Chakra, is the second energy center in the subtle body, located just below the navel and above the pubic bone. The term "Swadhisthana" translates from Sanskrit as "one's own abode" or "the dwelling place of the self." This chakra is the seat of our emotions, creativity, and sensuality, embodying our capacity for pleasure and interpersonal relationships.

The Swadhisthana Chakra is connected to the water element (Apas Tattva), which signifies fluidity, adaptability, and the emotional currents within us. A balanced Swadhisthana Chakra fosters a sense of emotional well-being, creativity, and healthy sexuality. When this chakra is imbalanced, we may experience issues related to emotional instability, creativity blocks, or unhealthy relationships.

Symbolism and Attributes

Swadhisthana Chakra / Sacral Chakra

- **Location:** Below the navel, above the pubic bone

- **Element:** Water (Apas Tattva)

- **Colour:** Orange (symbolizing creativity, enthusiasm, and emotional energy)

- **Shape:** Crescent Moon (representing fluidity and adaptability)

- **Petals:** Six (representing the dynamic and multifaceted nature of emotions)

- **Bija Mantra:** "Vam" (वं)

- **Deity:** Bhagwan Varuna (the god of water) and Mata Lakshmi (the goddess of abundance and prosperity)

- **Animal Symbol:** Crocodile (symbolizing primal instincts and adaptability)

- **Yantra:** A crescent moon within a circle, symbolizing the fluid nature of emotions

- **Sense:** Taste (associated with the water element and emotional expression)

- **Associated Planet:** Budh, Mercury

- **Mudra:** Varuna Mudra (Water Mudra)

Swadhisthana Chakra in Indian Tradition

In Indian tradition, the Swadhisthana Chakra is symbolized by an orange lotus with six petals, representing the dynamic nature of this energy center.

The colour orange is associated with vitality, enthusiasm, and the flow of creative energy.

The Swadhisthana Chakra is revered in Indian spiritual practices as the centre of emotional fluidity and creative expression.

It is linked to the flow of life's currents, akin to the river that adapts to its surroundings while continually moving forward.

In Vedic and Tantric traditions, this chakra is considered the source of creative power, and its energy is essential for artistic expression, joyful living, and fulfilling relationships.

Mata Lakshmi, the goddess of wealth and abundance, is often associated with the Swadhisthana Chakra. She embodies the flow of prosperity and the beauty of creativity.

Varuna, the god of water, represents the fluid and adaptable qualities of this chakra, emphasizing the importance of embracing change and maintaining emotional balance.

Before beginning the meditation practice, take a moment to learn Varun Mudra, a powerful hand gesture associated with the **Swadhisthana** Chakra.

Forming the Mudra

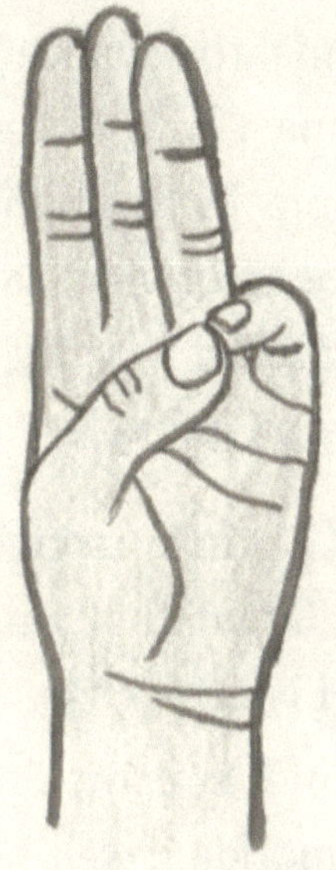

Varun Mudra

To form this mudra, touch the tip of your little finger (which represents the water element) to the tip of your thumb. Keep the other three fingers extended and relaxed. Rest your hands on your knees with palms facing upward.

Swadhisthana Chakra Meditation

Preparation: Find a quiet and serene space where you can meditate without disturbance. Choose a comfortable seated position, such as

Sukhasana (Easy Pose) or Vajrasana (Thunderbolt Pose), with your back straight. You may use an orange cloth or mat to enhance your connection to the Swadhisthana Chakra. Keep your hands in Anjali Mudra (prayer position) at the centre of your chest. Place an orange cloth or mat beneath you to further connect with the grounding energy of the Mooladhara Chakra.

Invocation: Begin by invoking the blessings of Mata Lakshmi. Chant the mantra: "Om Shreem Mahalakshmiyei Namaha" (ॐ श्रीमहालक्ष्मये नमः) to seek her guidance and support in enhancing your creativity and emotional well-being. Visualize her divine form, showering you with abundant, flowing energy.

Mudra and Pranayama

Hold Varun Mudra with both hands and practice **Sheetkari** Pranayama (Cooling Breath) by clenching your teeth and placing the tongue against the teeth.

Inhale slowly through the gaps between your teeth, feeling the cool, moist breath infuse your body with the soothing qualities of water. Close your mouth and exhale gently through your nose. With each inhalation, visualize yourself drawing in the refreshing moisture from the air, and with each exhalation, feel your mind calming down, releasing any emotional turbulence. Repeat this process for 5–10 rounds, focusing on the cooling sensation and relaxing any tension in the body.

Chanting the Bija Mantra: Maintaining the mudra start chanting the bija mantra "Vam" (वं) aloud or silently. Allow the sound to resonate in your lower abdomen, focus on the area below your navel, where the Swadhisthana Chakra is located. Visualize the orange lotus spinning gently, its six petals unfurling, opening with each chant. Feel the vibrations enhancing your creative expression and emotional fluidity. Imagine the lotus being nourished by the flowing waters of a serene river, symbolizing the fluid and dynamic nature of this chakra. Feel the flow of water energy rising through your body, bringing creativity and emotional balance.

Visualization of Yantra: To deepen your connection with the Swadhisthana Chakra, envision the crescent moon yantra at the center of this chakra, representing the fluidity and adaptability of your emotions. Feel the balancing of your emotional and creative energies.

Closing the Meditation: As you prepare to conclude, see the Swadhisthana Chakra glowing with steady, vibrant energy, spreading warmth and fluidity throughout your being. Slowly bring your awareness back to your breath, inhale and exhale deeply. Gently open your eyes and take a moment to feel the effects of the meditation. You may place your hands on your lower abdomen and offer a silent prayer of gratitude for the nurturing energy of the Swadhisthana Chakra.

Reflecting on the Experience: After your meditation, take some time to reflect on how you feel in terms of creativity, emotional balance, and adaptability. Be aware of insights or sensations that rise during the practice. This reflection can deepen your understanding of the Swadhisthana Chakra and its impact on your life.

Benefits of Swadhisthana Meditation

- **Emotional Well-Being:** Enhances emotional balance, reduces anxiety, and fosters a sense of joy and pleasure.

- **Creative Flow:** Stimulates creative expression and innovation, encouraging artistic endeavours and personal projects.

- **Healthy Relationships:** Promotes healthy, fulfilling relationships by improving emotional connectivity and openness.

- **Flexibility and Adaptability:** Increases your ability to adapt to changes and navigate life's challenges with ease.

Conclusion

The Swadhisthana Chakra is the wellspring of our emotional and creative life. By nurturing this chakra through meditation, chanting, mudra practice, and daily creative activities, we can foster a deep sense of emotional fluidity, creativity, and joy. This balanced energy center supports our ability to experience life fully, embrace change, and build fulfilling relationships. As we align the Swadhisthana Chakra, we enhance our overall well-being and open ourselves to the abundant flow of life's creative energies.

Manipura (Solar) Chakra

The Center of Personal Power and Transformation

Introduction to Manipura Chakra

The Manipura Chakra, often referred to as the Solar Plexus Chakra, is the third energy center in the subtle body, located in the area above the navel and below the chest.

The term "Manipura" translates from Sanskrit as "city of jewels" or "lustrous gem," symbolizing the radiant and transformative energy of this chakra. It is the seat of personal power, confidence, and the fire of transformation.

A balanced Manipura Chakra empowers us to pursue our goals with confidence, make decisive actions, and harness our personal power.

When this chakra is imbalanced, we may experience issues related to low self-esteem, lack of motivation, or difficulties in taking control of our lives.

Symbolism and Attributes

Manipura Chakra / Solar Plexus Chakra

- **Location:** Above the navel, below the chest

- **Element:** Fire (Agni Tattva)

- **Colour:** Yellow (symbolizing clarity, intellect, and personal power)

- **Shape:** Triangle (representing the fire element and the transformative energy)

- **Petals:** Ten (representing the aspects of personal strength and transformation)

- **Bija Mantra:** "Ram" (रं)

- **Deity:** Agni (the god of fire) and Surya (the sun god)

- **Animal Symbol:** Ram (symbolizing strength and courage)

- **Yantra:** A downward-pointing triangle within a circle, representing the transformative power of fire

- **Sense:** Sight (associated with clarity and perception)

- **Associated Planet:** Surya, Sun (representing vitality, authority, and self-expression)

- **Mudra:** Rudra Mudra (for personal power and transformation)

Manipura Chakra in Indian Tradition

In Indian tradition, the Manipura Chakra is symbolized by a yellow lotus with ten petals, representing the power and vibrancy of this energy center. The colour yellow is associated with clarity, intellect, and the fiery energy of transformation.

The Manipura Chakra is revered in Indian spiritual practices as the source of personal power and transformation. It is often compared to a blazing fire that transforms raw potential into manifested reality.

In Vedic and Tantric traditions, this chakra is essential for cultivating personal strength, ambition, and the ability to create change in one's life.

The Manipura Chakra is connected to the fire element (Agni Tattva), Agni, the god of fire, represents the transformative and purifying qualities of the Manipura Chakra.

Surya, the sun god, embodies the light and energy that this chakra radiates, enhancing vitality and self-confidence.

The downward-pointing triangle in the yantra symbolizes the harnessing of fiery energy for personal empowerment and transformation.

Before beginning the meditation practice, take a moment to learn Rudra Mudra, a powerful hand gesture associated with the **Manipura** Chakra.

Forming the Mudra

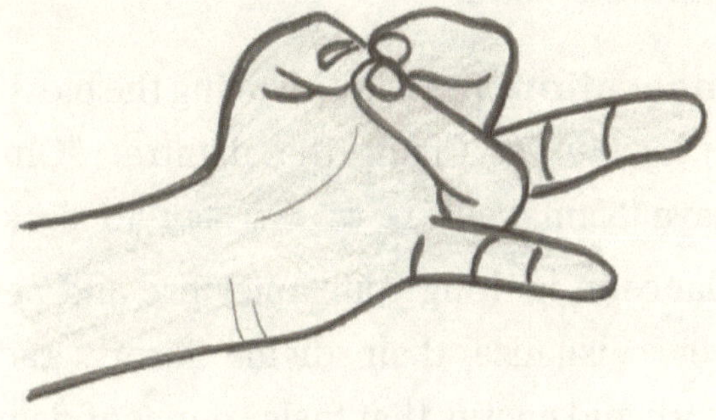

Rudra Mudra

To form this mudra, touch the tips of your thumb, index finger, and ring finger together, keeping the middle and little fingers extended. Rest your hands on your knees with palms facing upward. This mudra helps in harnessing personal power and transforming energy.

Manipura Chakra Meditation

Preparation: Choose a serene and quiet space for meditation. Sit in a comfortable seated position, such as Padmasana (Lotus Pose) or Sukhasana (Easy Pose), with your back straight and shoulders relaxed. Keep your hands in Anjali Mudra (prayer position) at the centre of your chest. Place a yellow cloth or mat beneath you to further connect with the grounding energy of the Manipura Chakra.

Invocation: Begin by invoking the blessings of Agni or Surya. Chant the mantra: "Om Ram Agnaye Namaha" (ॐ राम अग्नये नमः) to seek their guidance in igniting your inner fire and personal power. Visualize their divine forms, radiating warmth and energy that fuels your confidence and strength.

Pranayama: Practice Kapalabhati Pranayama (Skull Shining Breath) to stimulate the Manipura Chakra. Inhale deeply through your nose, then exhale forcefully through your nose, engaging your abdominal muscles. As you exhale, imagine releasing any self-doubt or stagnant energy. With each breath, visualize the fire of the Manipura Chakra burning brightly and transforming your energy.

Mudra and chanting the Bija Mantra: Now Hold Rudra Mudra with both hands and start chanting the bija mantra "Ram" (रं) aloud or silently. Allow the sound to resonate in your solar plexus, activating and harmonizing the Manipura Chakra. Visualize a bright yellow lotus with ten petals blooming in this area. Visualize the yellow lotus spinning and radiating with each chant fuelled by its vibrant energy. Feel the energy of confidence, power, and transformation filling you.

Visualization of Yantra: Maintain your awareness in the area just above your navel, where the Manipura Chakra is located. Envision the downward-pointing triangle yantra at the center of this chakra, representing the dynamic and transformative power of fire.

Closing the Meditation: As you complete your meditation, feel the bloomed yellow lotus of the Manipura Chakra spinning harmoniously, spreading its transformative energy expanding throughout your body. Slowly bring your awareness back to your breath, taking deep, invigorating inhales and exhales. Gently open your eyes and take a moment to feel the effects of the meditation. You may place your hands on your solar plexus and offer a silent prayer of gratitude for the empowering energy of the Manipura Chakra.

Reflecting on the Experience: After your meditation, take some time to reflect on how you feel in terms of personal power, clarity, and motivation. Be aware of insights or sensations that arise during the practice. This reflection can deepen your understanding of the Manipura Chakra and its impact on your life.

Benefits of Manipura Meditation

- **Personal Empowerment:** Enhances self-confidence, willpower, and the ability to take decisive action.

- **Clarity and Focus:** Improves mental clarity and focus, aiding in goal-setting and achievement.

- **Transformation:** Facilitates personal growth and transformation, helping you embrace change and overcome challenges.

- **Vitality and Strength:** Boosts physical energy and vitality, supporting overall health and well-being.

Conclusion

The Manipura Chakra is the center of our personal power and transformative energy. By nurturing this chakra through meditation, chanting, mudra practice, and daily actions, we can cultivate confidence, clarity, and the ability to manifest our goals. This balanced energy center empowers us to take control of our lives, embrace transformation, and live with purpose and vitality. As we align the Manipura Chakra, we enhance our overall strength and clarity, igniting the fire of our personal power.

ANAHATA (HEART) CHAKRA

The Center of Love and Compassion

Introduction to Anahata Chakra

The Anahata Chakra, also known as the Heart Chakra, is the fourth energy center in the subtle body, located in the center of the chest, near the heart.

The term "Anahata" translates from Sanskrit as "unstruck" or "unbeaten," symbolizing the pure, unconditional love and inner harmony that emanates from this chakra. It is the center of compassion, love, and emotional balance.

The Anahata Chakra is connected to the air element (Vayu Tattva), which signifies the flow of life, freedom, and the breath of life. A balanced Anahata Chakra fosters emotional well-being, compassion, and the ability to form meaningful connections with others. When this chakra is imbalanced, we may experience issues related to loneliness, difficulty in forming relationships, or emotional distress.

Symbolism and Attributes

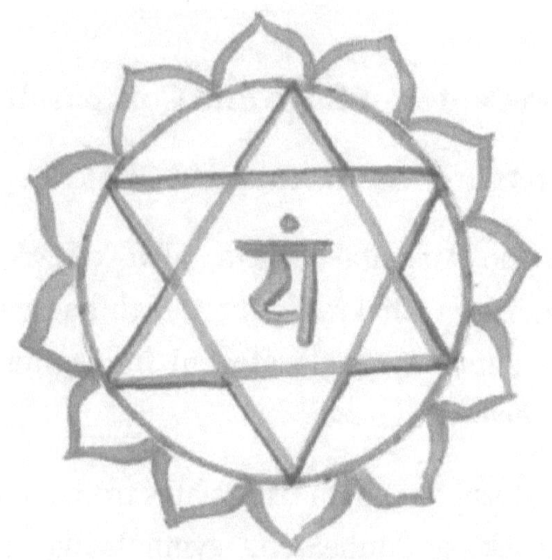

Anahata Chakra / Heart Chakra

- **Location:** Center of the chest, near the heart

- **Element:** Air (Vayu Tattva)

- **Color:** Green (symbolizing healing, growth, and unconditional love)

- **Shape:** Six-pointed star (representing the union of the physical and spiritual realms)

- **Petals:** Twelve (representing the qualities of love, empathy, and balance)

- **Bija Mantra:** "Yam" (यं)

- **Deity:** Bhagwan Shiv and Mata Parvati

- **Animal Symbol:** Antelope (symbolizing gentleness and peace)

- **Yantra:** A six-pointed star (Shatkona) within a circle, symbolizing the harmonious balance of energy

- **Sense:** Touch (associated with the feeling of connection and touch)

- **Associated Planet:** Chandra, Moon

- **Mudra:** Anahata Mudra (Heart Mudra)

Anahata Chakra in Indian Tradition

In Indian tradition, the Anahata Chakra is symbolized by a green lotus with twelve petals, representing the expansive and nurturing nature of this energy center.

The color green is associated with healing, growth, and the nurturing aspects of love. The Anahata Chakra governs our ability to give and receive love, cultivate empathy, and create harmonious relationships.

The Anahata Chakra is revered in Indian spiritual practices as the center of unconditional love and compassion.

It represents the divine essence of love that transcends personal desires and connects us to the universal whole.

In Vedic and Tantric traditions, this chakra is considered the bridge between the lower, more material aspects of our being and the higher, spiritual realms.

Ishvara, the lord of compassion, and Parvati, the goddess of love, are closely associated with the Anahata Chakra.

Their divine presence symbolizes the nurturing, healing, and loving qualities of this chakra. The six-pointed star yantra represents the balance and integration of the dual aspects of existence, symbolizing the harmonious flow of love and energy.

Before beginning the meditation practice, take a moment to learn Anahata Mudra, a powerful hand gesture associated with the Anahata Chakra.

Forming the Mudra

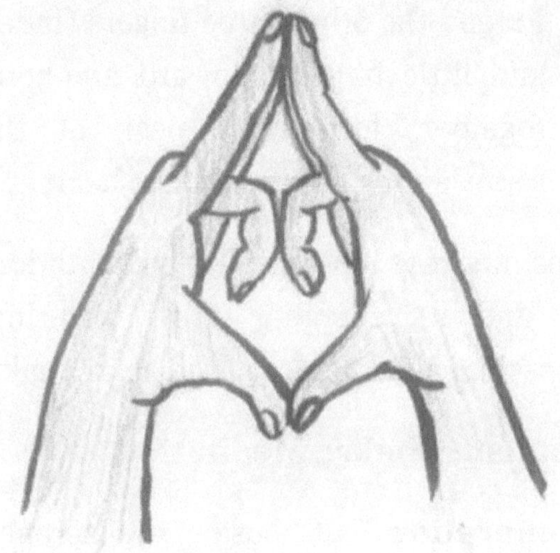

Anahata Mudra

- Bring your hands together at your heart center in a prayer position (Namaste).

- Gently open your palms away from each other, keeping the tips of your fingers touching.

- Place the backs of your middle fingers together and lower them towards the ground and your wrists, symbolizing the septum of the heart.

- Keep the pads of your thumbs touching.

- Extend the other three fingers (index, ring, and little fingers) upward and join them together, forming a peak at the top, representing the apex of the heart.

This mudra is a beautiful representation of the heart and its energetic flow, fostering love, compassion, and balance in the heart chakra.

Anahata Chakra Meditation

Preparation: Choose a serene and comfortable space for meditation. Sit in a relaxed seated position, such as Sukhasana (Easy Pose) or Padmasana (Lotus Pose), with your back straight and shoulders relaxed. Keep your hands in Anjali Mudra (prayer position) at the centre of your chest. Place a green cloth or mat beneath you to further connect with the grounding energy of the **Anahata** Chakra.

Invocation: Begin by invoking the blessings of Ishvara and Parvati. Chant the mantra: "Om Yam Ishvaraya Namaha" (ॐ यं ईश्वराय नमः) to seek their guidance in opening your heart to unconditional love and compassion. Visualize their divine forms, radiating love and healing energy that envelops your entire being.

Chanting the Bija Mantra: Form Anahata mudra and start chanting the bija mantra "Yam" (यं) aloud or silently. Allow the sound to resonate in your heart center, activating and harmonizing the Anahata Chakra. Visualize a vibrant green lotus with twelve petals blooming in this area and slowly spinning and radiating with each chant filling the energy of love, compassion, and emotional balance in your heart.

Pranayama for Anahata: Chandra Bhedana Pranayama, also known as Left Nostril Breathing, involves inhaling through the left nostril and exhaling through the right. This practice activates the **Ida nadi**, which is associated with the moon's cooling, calming energy. When Chandra Bhedana is practiced, it helps to calm the mind and regulate emotions, creating the inner peace necessary for the heart chakra to open and expand. It supports healing and fostering feelings of love and compassion.

Visualization of Yantra: To deepen your connection with the Anahata Chakra, envision the six-pointed star yantra at the center of this chakra, symbolizing the harmonious balance of love and energy. Feel their divine presence nurturing and healing your heart.

Closing the Meditation: As you conclude your meditation, visualize the green lotus of the Anahata Chakra spinning harmoniously, its petals radiating warmth and love. Slowly bring your awareness back to your breath, taking deep, soothing inhales and exhales. Gently open your eyes and take a moment to feel the effects of the meditation. You may place your hands on your heart and offer a silent prayer of gratitude for the loving energy of the Anahata Chakra.

Reflecting on the Experience: After your meditation, take some time to reflect on how you feel in terms of love, compassion, and emotional balance. Be aware of insights or sensations that arise during the practice. This reflection can deepen your understanding of the Anahata Chakra and its impact on your life.

Benefits of Anahata Meditation

- **Emotional Balance:** Enhances emotional stability, reduces stress, and fosters inner peace.

- **Compassion and Empathy:** Cultivates deeper compassion and empathy for others, improving relationships.

- **Heart Healing:** Promotes healing of emotional wounds and past hurts, facilitating forgiveness and self-love.

- **Connection and Harmony:** Strengthens your connection to others and creates harmonious interactions.

Conclusion

The Anahata Chakra is the center of our capacity for love, compassion, and emotional harmony.

By nurturing this chakra through meditation, chanting, mudra practice, and daily acts of kindness, we can cultivate a profound sense of connection and inner peace.

This balanced energy center enhances our ability to give and receive love, creating meaningful relationships and fostering a harmonious life.

As we align the Anahata Chakra, we open ourselves to the divine essence of love and compassion, enriching our overall well-being and emotional fulfillment.

Vishuddha (Throat) Chakra

The Center of Communication and Truth

Introduction to Vishuddha Chakra

The Vishuddha Chakra, also known as the Throat Chakra, is the fifth energy center in the subtle body, located in the region of the throat and neck.

The term "Vishuddha" translates from Sanskrit as "purification," reflecting the chakra's role in expressing our authentic voice and communicating with clarity and honesty. It is the center of verbal expression, truth, and self-expression.

The Vishuddha Chakra is connected to the ether element (Akasha Tattva), which signifies space, sound, and the medium through which our words and ideas resonate. A balanced Vishuddha Chakra fosters clear communication, creativity, and the courage to speak truthfully. When this chakra is imbalanced, we may experience issues related to fear of speaking, miscommunication, or a sense of being unheard.

Symbolism and Attributes

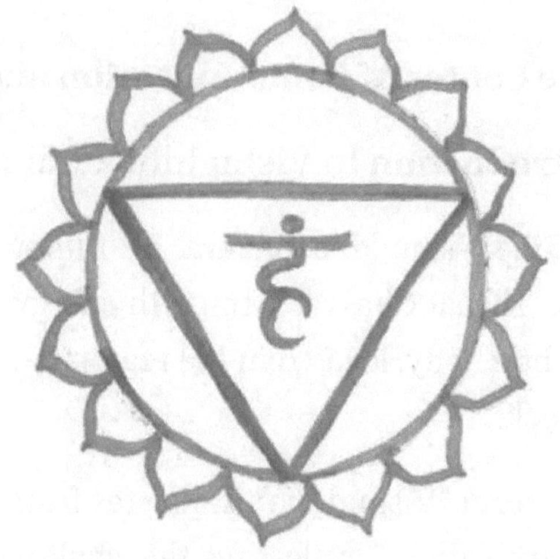

Vishuddha Chakra / Throat Chakra

- **Location:** Throat and neck region

- **Element:** Ether (Akasha Tattva)

- **Colour:** Turquoise Blue (symbolizing communication, wisdom, and purity)

- **Shape:** Circle (representing the space and the medium of sound)

- **Petals:** Sixteen (representing the power of expression and the expansion of consciousness)

- **Bija Mantra:** "Ham" (हं)

- **Deity:** Saraswati (the goddess of knowledge and wisdom) and Vishnu (the preserver of cosmic order)

- **Animal Symbol:** Elephant (symbolizing strength in communication and wisdom)

- **Yantra:** A circle with a central point (Bindu), symbolizing the essence of sound and purity

- **Sense:** Hearing (associated with listening and verbal expression)

- **Associated Planet:** Brihaspati, Jupiter

- **Mudra:** Vishuddha mudra

Vishuddha Chakra in Indian Tradition

In Indian tradition, the Vishuddha Chakra is symbolized by a turquoise blue lotus with sixteen petals, representing the purity and expansive nature of this energy center. The colour blue is associated with communication, wisdom, and the ability to speak one's truth. The Vishuddha Chakra governs our ability to articulate our thoughts, express our emotions, and communicate effectively with others.

The Vishuddha Chakra is revered in Indian spiritual practices as the center of purification and clear expression. It represents the power of the spoken word and the ability to communicate our inner truth. In Vedic and Tantric traditions, this chakra is considered crucial for expressing our authentic self and connecting with others through meaningful communication.

Saraswati, the goddess of knowledge, and Vishnu, the preserver of cosmic order, are closely associated with the Vishuddha Chakra. Their divine presence symbolizes the purity, wisdom, and clarity of expression that this chakra embodies. The circle yantra represents the space through which our words and ideas resonate, signifying the expansive nature of communication.

Before beginning the meditation practice, take a moment to learn Vishuddha mudra, a powerful hand gesture associated with the **Vishuddhi** Chakra.

Forming the Mudra

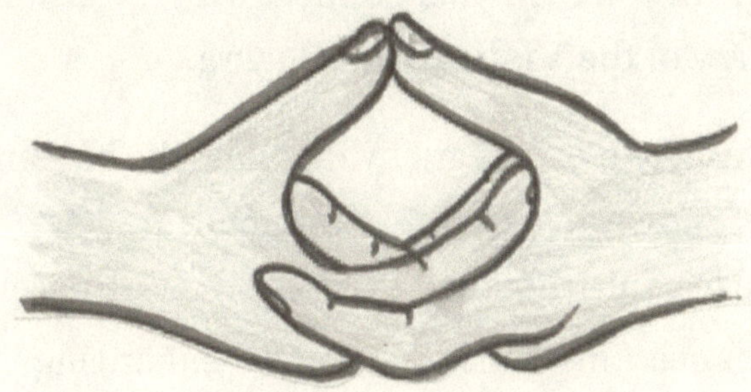

Vishuddha mudra

- Sit comfortably with your back straight.

- Place your hands near your chest, palms facing up.

- Interlock the fingers inside the palm.

- Press the tips of the thumbs against each other.

Vishuddha Chakra Meditation

1. Preparation: Find a quiet and serene space where you can meditate without disturbance. Choose a comfortable seated position, such as Sukhasana (Easy Pose) or Vajrasana (Thunderbolt Pose), with your back straight. Keep your hands in Anjali Mudra (prayer position) at the centre of your chest. Place a turquoise blue cloth or mat beneath you to further connect with the grounding energy of the **Vishuddha** Chakra.

Invocation: Begin by invoking the blessings of Ma Saraswati. Chant the mantra: "Om Ham Sarasvatyai Namaha" (ॐ हं सरस्वतये नमः) to seek her guidance in purifying and enhancing your communication abilities. Visualize her divine form, radiating clarity and wisdom that envelops your throat center.

Chanting the Bija Mantra: Form Vishuddha mudra and start chanting the bija mantra "Ham" (हं) aloud or silently. Allow the sound to resonate in your throat center, activating and harmonizing the Vishuddha Chakra. Visualize a vibrant turquoise blue lotus with sixteen petals blooming in this area see it spinning and radiating with each chant. Feel the energy of clear communication, truth, and self-expression filling you.

Pranayama for Vishuddha: Practice Ujjayi Pranayama (Victorious Breath) to stimulate the Vishuddha Chakra. Inhale deeply through your nose, slightly constricting your throat to create a soft sound, and exhale slowly with the same gentle sound. Visualize the breath as a purifying and expansive force that opens and balances the throat center. With each breath, imagine the energy of communication and clarity flowing freely.

Visualization of Yantra: To deepen your connection with the Vishuddha Chakra, envision the circle yantra with a central point (Bindu) at the center of this chakra, symbolizing the purity and essence of sound and expression. Feel the divine presence purifying and enhancing your ability to communicate.

Closing the Meditation: As you conclude your meditation, visualize its pure energy expanding throughout your throat. Slowly bring your awareness back to your breath, taking deep, soothing inhales and exhales. Gently open your eyes and take a moment to feel the effects of the meditation. You may place your hands on your throat and offer a silent prayer of gratitude for the purifying energy of the Vishuddha Chakra.

Reflecting on the Experience: After your meditation, take some time to reflect on how you feel in terms of communication, clarity, and self-expression. Be aware of insights or sensations that arise during the practice. This reflection can deepen your understanding of the Vishuddha Chakra and its impact on your life.

Benefits of Vishuddha Meditation:

- **Clear Communication:** Enhances your ability to express yourself clearly and effectively.

- **Authenticity:** Fosters honesty and authenticity in your interactions with others.

- **Emotional Release:** Helps in releasing fears and blockages related to self-expression.

- **Creative Expression:** Boosts creativity and the ability to articulate ideas and thoughts.

Conclusion

The Vishuddha Chakra is the center of our ability to communicate, express truth, and connect with others through authentic dialogue. By nurturing this chakra through meditation, chanting, mudra practice, and daily communication practices, we can cultivate clarity, honesty, and effective expression. This balanced energy center empowers us to speak our truth, listen deeply, and create meaningful connections. As we align the Vishuddha Chakra, we enhance our overall communication skills and embrace the purity of our authentic voice.

AJNA (THIRD EYE) CHAKRA

The Center of Intuition and Insight

Introduction to Ajna Chakra

The Ajna Chakra, also known as the Third Eye Chakra, is the sixth energy center in the subtle body, located in the center of the forehead, slightly above the space between the eyebrows.

The term "Ajna" translates from Sanskrit as "command" or "perceive," reflecting the chakra's role in intuition, insight, and inner vision. It is the center of higher perception, wisdom, and spiritual awareness.

The Ajna Chakra is connected to the mind element (Manas Tattva), which signifies the realm of thoughts, perception, and inner vision. A balanced Ajna Chakra fosters clarity of thought, intuitive insight, and spiritual understanding. When this chakra is imbalanced, we may experience issues related to confusion, lack of direction, or difficulty in connecting with our inner guidance.

Symbolism and Attributes

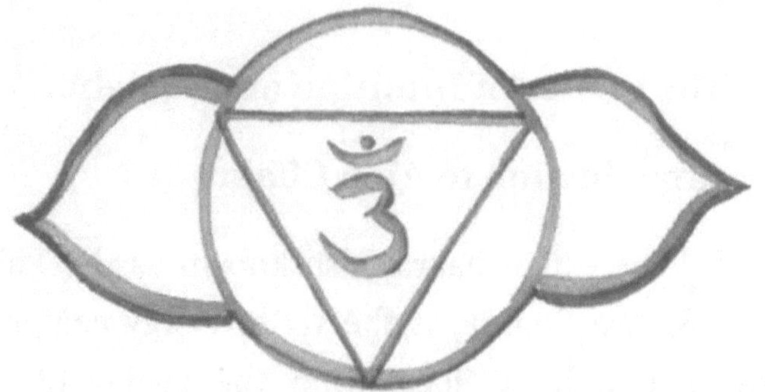

Ajna Chakra / Third Eye Chakra

- **Location:** Center of the forehead, between the eyebrows

- **Element:** Mind (Manas Tattva)

- **Color:** Indigo (symbolizing intuition, wisdom, and spiritual insight)

- **Shape:** Two-petaled lotus (representing duality and unity)

- **Petals:** Two (representing the balance of dual forces and higher perception)

- **Bija Mantra:** "Om" (ॐ)

- **Deity:** Shiva (the supreme consciousness) and Shakti (the divine energy)

- **Animal Symbol:** Elephant (symbolizing wisdom and clarity)

- **Yantra:** A two-petaled lotus with a central bindu, symbolizing the essence of higher consciousness and inner vision

- **Sense:** Sight (associated with inner vision and intuitive insight)

- **Associated Planet:** Shani, Saturn

- **Mudra:** Hakini Mudra (for concentration and intuition)

Ajna Chakra in Indian Tradition

In Indian tradition, the Ajna Chakra is symbolized by an indigo lotus with two petals, representing the balance between the material and spiritual realms.

The colour indigo is associated with intuition, insight, and the ability to see beyond the physical world. The Ajna Chakra governs our capacity for perception, inner knowing, and the ability to connect with higher consciousness.

The Ajna Chakra is highly revered in Indian spiritual practices as the center of higher perception and intuition.

It represents the power of inner vision and the ability to access deeper layers of consciousness. In Vedic and Tantric traditions, this chakra is considered crucial for spiritual awakening and understanding the true nature of reality.

Shiva, the supreme consciousness, and Shakti, the divine energy, are closely associated with the Ajna Chakra.

Their divine presence symbolizes the unity of consciousness and matter and the awakening of inner wisdom.

The two-petaled lotus yantra represents the balance between dual forces and the attainment of higher insight.

Before beginning the meditation practice, take a moment to learn Hakini Mudra, a powerful hand gesture associated with the **Ajna** Chakra.

Forming the Mudra

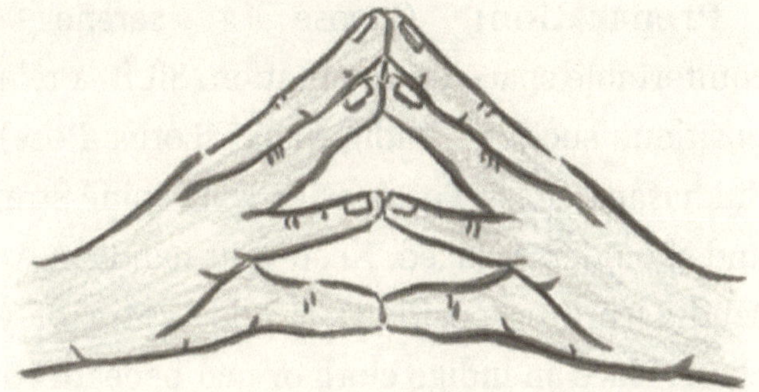

Hakini Mudra

- Sit comfortably with your back straight.

- Bring your hands to chest level, palms facing each other.

- Touch the tips of all five fingers on your right hand to the corresponding fingertips on your left hand.

- Keep the palms slightly apart, creating a hollow space between them.

- Ensure the fingertips remain gently touching, with the fingers forming an arch or dome shape.

Ajna Chakra Meditation

Preparation: Choose a serene and comfortable space for meditation. Sit in a relaxed position, such as Padmasana (Lotus Pose) or Sukhasana (Easy Pose), with your spine straight and shoulders relaxed. Keep your hands in Anjali Mudra (prayer position) at the centre of your chest. Place an indigo cloth or mat beneath you to further connect with the grounding energy of the **Ajna** Chakra.

Invocation: Begin by invoking the blessings of Shiva and Shakti. Chant the mantra: "Om Namah Shivaya" (ॐ नमः शिवाय) to seek their guidance in awakening your inner vision and intuitive insight. Visualize their divine forms, radiating indigo light that envelops your forehead and enhances your spiritual awareness.

Chanting the Bija Mantra: Form Hakini mudra and start chanting the bija mantra "Om" (ॐ) aloud or silently. Allow the sound to resonate in your forehead center, activating and harmonizing the Ajna Chakra. Visualize the indigo lotus spinning and radiating with each chant. Feel the energy of intuitive insight and spiritual awareness filling you.

Pranayama for Ajna: Practice Nadi Shodhana Pranayama (Alternate Nostril Breathing) to enhance the flow of energy to the Ajna Chakra. Inhale deeply through your left nostril, hold the breath briefly, and exhale slowly through your right nostril. Alternate the process, visualizing the breath as a cleansing and balancing force that opens and harmonizes the third eye center. With each breath, imagine the energy of clarity and insight flowing freely.

Visualization of Yantra: To deepen your connection with the Ajna Chakra, bring your awareness to the center of your forehead, where the Ajna Chakra is located. Envision the two-petaled lotus yantra with a central bindu at the center of this chakra, symbolizing the essence of higher consciousness and inner vision. Feel their divine presence guiding and awakening your intuitive insight.

Closing the Meditation: As you conclude your meditation, visualize the indigo lotus of the Ajna Chakra spinning harmoniously, its petals radiating with clarity and insight. Slowly bring your awareness back to your breath, taking deep, soothing inhales and exhales. Gently open your eyes and take a moment to feel the effects of the meditation. You may place your hands on your forehead and offer a silent prayer of gratitude for the awakening of your inner vision.

Reflecting on the Experience: After your meditation, take some time to reflect on how you feel in terms of intuition, insight, and spiritual awareness. Be aware of insights or sensations that arise during the practice. This reflection can deepen your understanding of the Ajna Chakra and its impact on your life.

Benefits of Ajna Meditation

- **Intuitive Clarity:** Enhances your ability to trust and follow your intuition.

- **Mental Clarity:** Improves clarity of thought and decision-making.

- **Spiritual Insight:** Fosters a deeper connection to spiritual wisdom and higher consciousness.

- **Inner Vision:** Strengthens the ability to see beyond the physical world and perceive deeper truths.

Conclusion

The Ajna Chakra is the center of our intuitive perception, spiritual insight, and inner vision. By nurturing this chakra through meditation, chanting, mudra practice, and daily mindfulness, we can cultivate a profound sense of clarity, wisdom, and spiritual awareness. This balanced energy center empowers us to trust our intuition, see beyond the physical realm, and connect with higher consciousness. As we align the Ajna Chakra, we enhance our overall understanding and embrace the depth of our inner vision.

Sahasrara (Crown) Chakra

The Center of Divine Connection and Enlightenment

Introduction to Sahasrara Chakra

The Sahasrara Chakra, also known as the Crown Chakra, is the seventh and final energy center in the subtle body, located at the top of the head. The term "Sahasrara" translates from Sanskrit as "thousand-petaled," symbolizing the vast, boundless nature of this chakra. It represents the pinnacle of spiritual consciousness and our connection to the divine and universal consciousness.

In Indian tradition, the Sahasrara Chakra is symbolized by a thousand-petaled lotus, often depicted in shades of violet or white. This lotus represents the infinite nature of spiritual enlightenment and the connection to the divine source. The color white or violet is associated with purity, spiritual awakening, and transcendence. The Sahasrara Chakra governs our ability to connect with higher consciousness, experience unity with the universe, and attain enlightenment.

The Sahasrara Chakra is connected to the divine or spiritual element (Paramatman Tattva), which signifies the supreme consciousness and the essence of being. A balanced Sahasrara Chakra fosters a profound sense of spiritual connection, inner peace, and enlightenment. When this chakra is imbalanced, we may experience feelings of disconnection, lack of purpose, or spiritual confusion.

Symbolism and Attributes

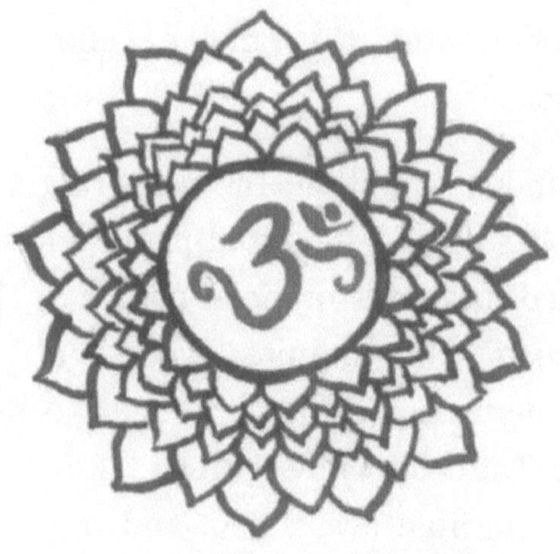

Sahasrara Chakra / Crown Chakra

- **Location:** Top of the head

- **Element:** Divine or Spiritual (Paramatman Tattva)

- **Color:** Violet or White (symbolizing purity, spiritual awakening, and transcendence)

- **Shape:** Thousand-petaled lotus (representing the infinite nature of divine consciousness)

- **Petals:** Thousand (representing the expansive and boundless nature of spiritual awareness)

- **Bija Mantra:** "Om" (ॐ)

- **Deity:** Brahman (the supreme cosmic spirit) and Shiva (the ultimate consciousness)

- **Animal Symbol:** None specific (symbolizing the transcendence of worldly forms)

- **Yantra:** A thousand-petaled lotus with a central bindu, symbolizing the essence of divine consciousness and unity

- **Sense:** Consciousness (associated with spiritual awareness and unity)

- **Associated Planet:** None specific (symbolizing transcendence beyond material influences)

- **Mudra:** Sahasrara Mudra (for divine connection and enlightenment)

Sahasrara Chakra in Indian Tradition

The Sahasrara Chakra is revered in Indian spiritual practices as the center of divine connection and ultimate enlightenment. It represents the culmination of spiritual growth and the realization of oneness with the divine. In Vedic and Tantric traditions, this chakra is considered the gateway to experiencing the highest states of consciousness and spiritual realization.

Brahman, the supreme cosmic spirit, and Shiva, the ultimate consciousness, are closely associated with the Sahasrara Chakra. Their divine presence symbolizes the unity of all existence and the attainment of spiritual enlightenment. The thousand-petaled lotus yantra represents the infinite and boundless nature of spiritual awareness and the realization of divine unity.

Before beginning the meditation practice, take a moment to learn Sahasrara Mudra, a powerful hand gesture associated with the Sahasrara Chakra.

Forming the Mudra

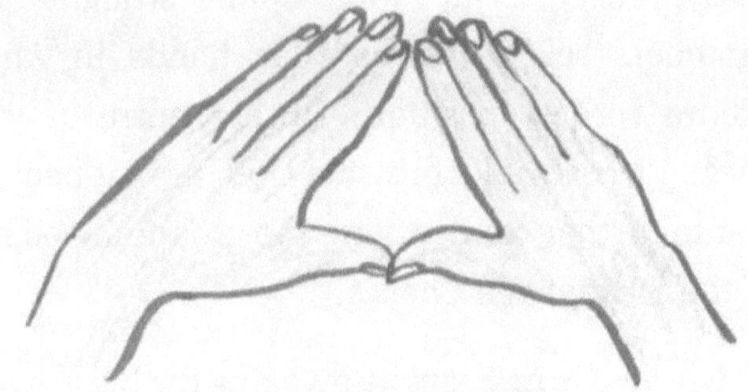

Sahasrara Mudra

- Sit comfortably with your back straight.

- Bring both hands in front of your chest.

- Touch the tips of your thumbs and index fingers together, forming a triangle.

- Keep the other fingers extended and relaxed, pointing upward.

- Hold this position gently, maintaining the triangular shape created by your thumbs and index fingers.

Sahasrara Chakra Meditation

Preparation: Find a tranquil and sacred space for meditation. Sit in a comfortable position, such as Padmasana (Lotus Pose) or Sukhasana (Easy Pose), with your spine straight and shoulders relaxed. Keep your hands in Anjali Mudra (prayer position) at the centre of your chest. Place a violet or white cloth or mat beneath you to further connect with the grounding energy of the **Sahasrara** Chakra.

Invocation: Begin by invoking the blessings of Brahman and Shiva. Chant the mantra: "Om Namah Shivaya" (ॐ नमः शिवाय) to seek their guidance in awakening your divine consciousness and spiritual insight. Visualize their divine forms, radiating white or violet light that envelops the top of your head and connects you to the infinite source of consciousness.

Chanting the Bija Mantra: Form Sahasrara mudra and start chanting the bija mantra "Om"

(ॐ) aloud or silently. Allow the sound to resonate at the top of your head, activating and harmonizing the Sahasrara Chakra. Visualize the thousand-petaled lotus spinning and radiating with each chant. Feel the energy of divine connection and enlightenment filling you.

Pranayama for Sahasrara: Practice Brahmari Pranayama (Bee Breath) to enhance the flow of energy to the Sahasrara Chakra. Inhale deeply through your nose, and as you exhale, produce a soft humming sound like a bee. Visualize the vibration of the sound as a divine resonance that opens and balances the crown center. With each breath, imagine the energy of spiritual awareness and unity flowing freely.

Visualization of Yantra: To deepen your connection with the Sahasrara Chakra, visualize Brahman and Shiva as radiant beings, their forms glowing with the white or violet light of the chakra. Envision the thousand-petaled lotus yantra with a central bindu at the center of this chakra, symbolizing the essence of divine consciousness and unity. Feel their divine presence guiding and awakening your spiritual awareness.

Closing the Meditation: As you conclude your meditation, visualize the thousand-petaled lotus of the Sahasrara Chakra spinning harmoniously, its petals radiating with divine light and unity. Slowly bring your awareness back to your breath, taking deep, soothing inhales and exhales. Gently open your eyes and take a moment to feel the effects of the meditation. You may place your hands on the top of your head and offer a silent prayer of gratitude for the awakening of your divine consciousness.

Reflecting on the Experience: After your meditation, take some time to reflect on how you feel in terms of spiritual connection, awareness, and enlightenment. Be aware of insights or sensations that rise during the practice. This reflection can deepen your understanding of the Sahasrara Chakra and its impact on your life.

Benefits of Sahasrara Meditation

- **Divine Connection:** Enhances your ability to connect with higher consciousness and the divine source.

- **Spiritual Enlightenment:** Fosters a profound sense of spiritual awareness and unity with the universe.

- **Inner Peace:** Promotes inner peace and serenity through the realization of divine essence.

- **Expanded Consciousness:** Strengthens the awareness of your true nature and the interconnectedness of all existence.

Conclusion

The Sahasrara Chakra is the center of our divine connection, spiritual enlightenment, and cosmic awareness. By nurturing this chakra through meditation, chanting, mudra practice, and daily spiritual practices, we can cultivate a profound sense of unity with the divine and the universe.

This balanced energy center empowers us to embrace the purity and expansiveness of our true self and realize our connection to the infinite source of consciousness.

As we align the Sahasrara Chakra, we open ourselves to the boundless wisdom and divine essence that resides within and around us.

DISCLAIMER

Please Note: Avoid the urge to practice all mudras and meditations at once. Begin by understanding the purpose of each mudra and chakra, and select one that addresses your current physical and emotional needs. Start with just a few minutes of practice, gradually increasing to around 20 minutes in one sitting.

For deeper pranic purification, longer practice periods may be beneficial but should only be undertaken under the strict guidance of a qualified Guru.

If you are experiencing any psychological disturbances, do not begin these meditations without proper consultation with both a Yoga Guru and your healthcare professional. Your well-being is paramount, and personalized guidance is essential for safe and effective practice.

ABOUT THE AUTHOR

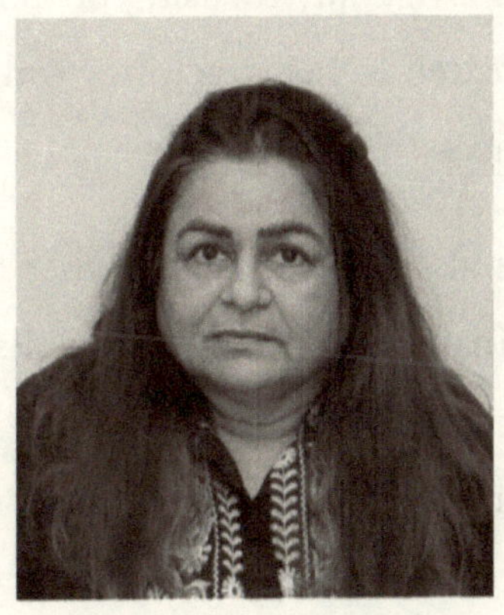

Shilpa Mehta: *A Journey of Yoga and Lifelong Learning*

Shilpa Mehta embarked on her Yoga journey in 1996, immersing herself in the true essence of Yoga at an ashram. Her practice deepened through training at esteemed institutions such as The Yoga Institute, Kaivalya Dham, Shri Ambika Yoga Kutir, and Mumbai University. During this period, she also taught Kathak dance and pre-primary classes, showcasing her versatility as an educator.

An avid reader, traveler, and YouTuber, Shilpa began sharing her Yoga expertise in 1998. Over the years, she has conducted various health camps for professionals, including doctors, executives, chartered accountants, and teachers. Originally focusing on physical platform, Shilpa now extends her teachings online, reaching a global audience.

Shilpa has also coordinated teacher training courses at The Yoga Institute for more than a decade. Holding a master's degree in philosophy and having studied positive psychology, she brings a deep intellectual and emotional understanding to her practice. Additionally, she has served as a speaker and judge at international Yoga conferences.

Currently, Shilpa teaches Yoga at Dhirubhai Ambani International School and has been dedicated to her craft for over 21 years. Her passion for Yoga not only ignites her purpose in life but also fulfills it through both practice and teaching.

MAY I ASK YOU FOR A SMALL FAVOR?

At the outset, I want to thank you for reading this book. You could have chosen any other book, but you took mine, and I appreciate this.

I hope you got at least a few actionable insights that will positively impact your day-to-day life.

Can I ask for 30 seconds more of your time?

I'd love it if you could leave a review of the book. That will help me grow my readership by encouraging folks to take a chance on my books.

Keeping it straight - reviews are the lifeblood of any author.

It will take less than a minute of your time but will help me reach out to more people.

If you enjoyed this book, I would greatly appreciate it if you could leave an honest review where you purchased it. I'd love to read your thoughts. Thank you for your support!

Mudras For Teachers: Enhance Voice Clarity, Cultivate Emotional Resilience, Boost Classroom Presence, and Empower Teaching With Hand Gestures